DMSO

A miracle drug

Contents

Introduction

Natural remedies and herbs have been used in traditional medicine for many centuries. Extracts from plants and trees have proved efficacious in treating many illnesses. DMSO or Dimethyl sulfoxide is one such natural product produced from bark of trees. DMSO is a byproduct of the paper manufacturing process. Some have called DMSO a miracle cure for many human ailments. It can be used alone or with combination with other drugs. Thousands of studies have been conducted to prove the efficacy of DMSO. It is predicted that Dimethyl sulfoxide has many other applications which are yet to be discovered. In this book you will read about the many wonder miracles and cures of DMSO or Dimethyl sulfoxide.

The medical world has been expanding at very fast pace. Medical intervention has created wonder drugs which can make you a god – flawless, healthy and young. Babies are being produced in test tubes. You no longer require being a woman to have your own baby. Surrogacy provides an alternate to women suffering from illnesses which deny them the opportunities to become a mother. There are miracle cures for heart attack and mental diseases.

DMSO has numerous properties which makes it a suitable medicine for many illnesses. It can also be found in nature in vast quantities. Loggers have been using DMSO for treating wounds. It can also be ingested without apparent side effects. Obviously, too much of anything is dangerous. Still there have been no known reports of DMSO overdosing. As new discoveries in medicine, especially in genetics and cancer treatment, scientists are looking for ways to accelerate the pace of drug development.

New discoveries are unraveling a host of medical solutions which benefit the human race. However, in the midst of plenty there is a silence on many natural substances which may provide alternate solutions to illnesses. DMSO is one such wonder drug which has remained under the radar for many years. There is no specific reason why DMSO has been neglected. Is it that big pharma companies fear that their multibillion dollar drug formulations may not find a market in case DMSO i9s found to be a cheaper alternative? There is no evidence to prove that pharmaceutical companies are deliberately underplaying the role of DMSO. In this book you will find many prospective cures with DMSO. Also, DMSO can be used in a non-medical setting as well. We will have a brief look at other uses of DMSO.

Chapter 1 - What is DMSO?

DMSO has been known for many years. In fact it was discovered in late nineteenth century Alexander Zaytsev, a Russian chemist. For a very long time the discovery did not find any practical use. This phenomenon of important discoveries not finding a place in the public domain is not uncommon. Initially industrial chemists tried to use it as a solvent because of its properties.

It is interesting to note that most practical applications of naturally occurring chemicals have been accidental. The same is the case with DMSO. Earlier, before the use of DSMO, transplant organs underwent ice crystallization at low temperature which killed the live tissues. Amazingly DMSO offered properties which allowed preservation of transplant organs in low temperature. It comes as no surprise that DMSO is still being used as a preservative for transplant organs at low temperature (though other ways have also been found).

This application in preserving transplant organs gave rise to a fresh interest in the palliative properties of

DMSO. Many scientific journals carried articles citing various remedies of DMSO. It must be noted that the exact mode of action by which DMSO works has still not been properly understood. DMSO is being used to cure numerous illnesses which cannot be treated with known allopathic medicines. One of the properties of DMSO is its distinctive odor of garlic. This makes double blind studies of DMSO difficult.

Chapter 2 - Applications and uses of DMSO

There has been a spurt in studies involving free radicals. It has been found that free radicals, when produced in the body, causes damage to healthy cells. Your body organ start deteriorating and behaving abnormally when exposed to free radicals. The damage caused by free radicals is slow and therefore difficult to detect, and by the time the damage is discovered it is usually too late. DMSO is known to remove the free radicals from the body. DMSO is also known to preserve your body's natural immune system.

DMSO has an interesting property of diffusing or permeating easily your skin. You will read about the various unique remedies using this property of DMSO throughout this book. In fact, DMSO dissolves so quickly into the skin that within no time the patient can taste garlic in his mouth.

The blood brain barrier

The blood–brain barrier plays an important part in protecting the brain from many diseases caused by bacteria, viruses and other pathogens. The blood–

brain barrier prevents selective transportation of pathogenic material from the blood to the brain. What this means I that your brain is protected and remain free from infection. However, this also creates problems when you have to transport medicines to the brain. The brain barrier does not allow medicines to reach the brain. This can prove to be a hindrance during treatment of mental illnesses. Though smart drugs have been developed, we still have a long way to go in achieving good penetrability of drugs to the brain. In this context the specific property of DMSO to penetrate the blood–brain barrier comes in handy. This property can be used to allow transportation of essential drugs to the brain. A similar behavior of DMSO is its vasodilatory property. Blood flow to injured organ becomes restricted when the blood vessels constrict. DMSO can improve blood flow to injured organs by dilating blood vessels leading to the affected are.

Why is DMSO or Dimethyl sulfoxide special? There are many reasons why DMSO can be considered to be a unique substance with curative properties. Of particular interest to scientists and medical practitioners is the ability to quickly get absorbed by the skin. This property can be gauged by the fact that application of DMSO on the skin almost immediately results in garlic taste in the mouth. Can this property be used to transport other medicines through the skin by mixing it with DMSO? Scientists certainly think so. Not only this, but the property of DMSO to provide protection to the nervous system, when injected, is also worth mentioning.

Many experiments have been conducted on animals to ascertain the benefits of DMSO. Interest in the subject has grown and a rash of conferences on DMSO proves that the scientific community hopes to find many valuable applications of DMSO in the medical domain.

Chemical compounds riding piggyback on DMSO

DMSO has been shown to play an important role in genetics. Genetic engineers have by now established that humans suffer from numerous diseases arising out of unhealthy mutation of genes. These mutations or changes occur spontaneously and their time and occurrence cannot be ascertained apriori(before their occurrence). For instance some proteins lack the ability to fold by themselves due to mutation occurring in the proteins of the affected cells. DMSO can be sued to assist in the folding of the damaged proteins.

DMSO as battery chemical

Witness the recent developments in electric cars and vehicles. The most important component in an electric car is the battery. There is hectic activity in the field of heavy duty, sustainable, light, long lasting and efficient batteries. You would be surprised to learn that DMSO acts as an efficient electrolyte in batteries. This property of DMSO is derived from its unique chemical structure.

DMSO for organ preservation

We have already touched upon this subject. However, due to the importance of this specific activity of DMSO, a more descriptive explanation is needed.

Organ transplants have now become a common medical practice. Healthy organs are removed from cadavers or from donors and placed in patients. The problem arises from there is a time lapse between removal of organ and placement in recipients patients. The healthy organs start deteriorating quickly in normal room temperature. The entire process can get negated due to the rotting of organs. These organs are therefore preserved or frozen in subzero temperatures. Cell deterioration can be arrested by freezing them. This seems simple enough. However, organ tissues contain water which freezes along with the organ itself. The frozen water forms ice crystals which damage the tissues and make them unusable. To overcome this problem, organs are kept in a medium which avoids crystallization. There are many preservants which are used and DMSO is one of them. Studies have shown that amount of DMSO required is considerably less as compared to other preservants. DMSO also causes less damage to the organ cells. It is also found to be less toxic.

Stem cells are extracted from umbilical cord and preserved for future use. These stem cells are intended for use at a later date if and when required. They may be used in case of accidents to the original donor or some such circumstances. . DMSO is a preservative of choice for such stem cells.

How does the body react to DMSO?

After administering DMSO, the blood, stools and urine of patients has been examined. This examination provides information on the rate of absorption of the DMSO, its metabolism and excretion properties. It has been observed that DMSO gets widely absorbed in tissues and fluids. It is excreted through urine, feces, breath and also the skin. DMSO can stay for a fortnight after administration.

DMSO for pain relief

Is there anyone who has not felt pain at some stage of life or other? Pain is the most common ailment for which we approach a physician. Pain may be a common affliction but its effect on our quality of life has been underestimated. But there is a reason why we feel pain. Imagine that you touch a hot bowl of soup and it scalds your fingers. The pain which you feel warns you against holding the bowl and you immediately drop it. As a result you save your fingers from getting burnt. The pain may still persist due to the swelling of the fingers. The tissues of the fingers have been hurt and they show their displeasure by sending signals of pain. Another type of pain is felt when there is an inflammation of tissues. This may happen due to injury or due to infection. Your movements get restricted till the pain subsides. The third type of pain can be called pathological, which arises due to persistent or intense stimuli. In all three cases, pain brings down your ability to lead a happy and healthy life.

You can end up dead while trying to get rid of pain in your body. Obviously this I not a joke, since according to a report written by the Centers for Disease Control and Prevention (CDC), many thousands of deaths occur due to use of opioids for pain control. Many of these deaths also happen due to use of opioids for recreational purposes. What this mean is that use of opioids for treating pain has the potential to be abused. Not surprisingly, there is a desperate search for alternate therapies for pain alleviation. DMSO seems to be an exciting alternative.

It should be noted that characterization of pain is a difficult task by itself. Quantifying the type of pain, its strength and the time period of its onslaught can be mind-blowingly tough.

The main advantage of using DMSO for pain relief is the fact that it is not habit forming. You can't get addicted to DMSO even after prolonged use. How does the pain relief mechanism of DMSO differ from that of an opioid? To ascertain whether there is a difference in the pain relieving mechanism, several experiments were conducted on rats. Why rats? Usually researchers prefer using rat as the experimental animal because its organs and behavior resemble closely with humans. The analgesic or pain relieving mechanism in rats was studied to understand the underlying process. Another question which required an explanation was whether DMSO was a analgesic at all and at what dosage. It does not make sense to use any substance as a medication if you have to consume enormous quantities to produce significant effect. The results of an experiment showed that DMSO did produce analgesic effect at large doses. DMSO moreover did not act as an anesthetic. The analgesic effect caused by morphine lasted around two hours while that by DMSO remained for twenty four hours. It was also observed that the analgesic effect produced by morphine and DMSO was different. This gave rise to another question? What was the mechanism used by DMSO if its pain relieving mechanism was not induced by blocking morphine receptors? Further research has been conducted and has led to several significant conclusions. One of them is that DMSO can be used effectively in relieving pain originating from musculoskeletal sources.

DMSO and anti-inflammation

We had touched upon lightly on this aspect of DMSO earlier. Inflammation is a localized reaction produced by the body when exposed to trauma. For example, you may twist your finger which can cause puffing of the finger joint. This protects the finger against damage and promotes release of chemicals which create a healing environment. Inflammation occurs in case of neuro and cardio diseases as well as in arthritis and bone related symptoms. However, inflammation and subsequent pain are only a symptom of a larger malice. Studies have shown that application of DMSO on the skin around the affected area produces significant reduction in inflammation, though the exact mechanism of operation could not be explained. It was opined that the prostaglandin pathways may have a role to play in the anti-inflammatory properties of DMSO.

DMSO and heart diseases

We are all familiar with the heart and the problems it creates in our lives. On the other hand we can't be heartless when love is in the air. In addition to the affair of the heart, we are also in danger of it stopping to function due to reasons other than jilted love.

Physically, our heart deals with blood and its flow. Impure blooded or deoxygenated blood enters the heart. Here oxygen from the lungs mixes with the blood and this is purified blood is pumped into our body. Though the process looks simple, many things can go wrong while the heart goes about doing its mundane task. Sometimes even death can occur due to a dysfunctional heart. One of the medical terms used in heart related diseases is myocardial infarction. Many experiments have been conducted to observe the effect of DMSO in treatment of myocardial infarction. In one such experiment it was observed that DMSO provided relief to rat's heart suffering from artificially induced injury by reoxygenation process. This process causes the blood flow in the heart to reduce. The heart also experiences excessive and abnormal contraction. When DMSO was introduced into the heart before reoxygenation, it was observed that it resulted in significant reduction in heart contraction. This lead scientists and researchers to conclude that DMSO could be used for reducing trauma caused to the heart due to reoxygenation. It was also noticed that DMSO facilitates flow of oxygen into the thick heart tissues which protects the heart from ischemia.

Heart attacks can occur due to narrowing of coronary vessels. The accumulation of platelets on the walls of the blood vessels reduce their size. Currently this condition is treated by dilating these blood vessels using various drugs. The role of DMSO as a deaggregator is important in such situations. In experiments using DMSO as a dissolving agent, it was observed that DMSO itself played the most important role as a deaggregator than the drug.

We have already discussed the property of DMSO as a scavenger. This property comes in handy when DMSO is used in treatment of heart diseases. Free radicals are produced more copiously during heart infarction and the normal secretion of chemicals and enzymes is unable to cope with the amount of free radicals. DMSO helps in coping with excess production of free radicals during injury to heart muscles.

Another interesting property of DMSO is its ability to work as a sodium channel blocker. Minerals such as sodium and calcium play an important role in maintaining the contractions of the heart. Any mismatch in the quantity of either of these minerals causes the heart to beat unevenly. DMSO inhibits the infusion of sodium and calcium into cells. Interestingly, DMSO prevents influx of sodium and calcium into cells but allows outflow of potassium from the cells. The results available after conducting experiments are not conclusive. Establishing the exact mechanism of operation of DMSO on ion balance will be of great significance to the study of heart conditions.

It is interesting to note that there I no other chemical or drug which combines all these properties of DMSO. Obviously, DMSO can play an important role in the field of cardiac surgery. DMSO's ability to inhibit blood clot formation can be used for treatment of ischemia. The ability to stop influx of sodium and calcium into cells gives it a unique ability to treat patients suffering from irregular heartbeat. As a scavenger of free radicals it can be utilized to maintain a healthy heart condition.

Use of DMSO in treating bowel inflammation

Isn't it surprising that even after advances in science and medicine there are still some ailments which have no explanation? Inflammatory bowel is one such affliction. It appears that the cause of inflammation is unknown. This condition is observed in patients developing diarrhea accompanied with blood. The occurrence of diarrhea is not periodical. The condition results in inflammation of the rectum and may include the entire colon. The patients do not enjoy total cure from this ailment and the focus of medical professionals is only restricted to reducing the inflammation with the use of anti-inflammatory drugs. These drugs contain steroids which has a direct impact on the normal functioning of patients. In the absence of any other cure, these patients have to endure the pain and other side effects which are a byproduct of treatment.

One of the novel approaches being tried is the use of DMSO as a free radical scavenger. It is opined that removal of free radicals from the inflammation site can prevent recurrence of attacks.

DMSO as penetrative agent

You may have noticed that not all drugs can penetrate the skin. Your skin can prove to be a serious soldier preventing the movement of illegal immigrants into the nation called your body. The skin forms a natural barrier or wall, if you wish to call it that, keeping external agents from entering the body. In a normal healthy body this is an enviable job, but when it comes to drug delivery through the skin, the same property can prove to be an irritant. What if you had a chemical which could easily and rapidly penetrate the skin? Perhaps this chemical could allow other drugs to piggy back and transport them across the cutaneous layer (skin). DMSO performs this task quite efficiently. Not only does DMSO penetrate the skin but it can also facilitate transport of other drugs across the skin barrier.

Some people have a thick skin. Some others have a soft skin. The people with tough leather are not affected by sudden cold or heat, while others may howl in pain. Drug penetration through the skin also depends on the thickness of the dermal layer which differs from person to person. Moreover, the penetration also depends on the diffusion ability of individual skin. The amount of drug penetration also depends on the quantity of the drug applied. Obviously a bottle of any given drug would be more effective than a mere spoon applied on the skin.

The problem is that you can't change the thickness of the skin to allow penetration of drug. The only way out is to use materials which can intrinsically get diffused into the skin. DMSO has shown promise in this area.

Healing properties of DMSO

At some point or other all of us have got hurt. The pain is insufferable and it takes a long time to heal the wounds. Who would not wish that there was a miracle cure for wounds? DMSO has shown remarkable improvement in reduction of pain and also faster healing of wounds. The healing process is quite complex. In the healing process a chemical is released by the body which though essential, must not be excessive. The balance in release is critical. DMSO assists in release of this chemical as well as limits the amount of discharge.

There are two types of wounds. The acute wound occurs when we have an accident. This type of wound is unlikely to occur at the same place again. On the other hands chronic wounds are those which occur when a patient suffers from ulcers and other skin related diseases. This cause inflammation of the affected area and may also be painful. Use of DMSO in such cases has been studied extensively. The results suggest that DMSO plays an important role in both healing wounds and alleviating pain. Moreover the toxicity of DMSO has been found to be low. Many wounds occur as a result of cancer treatment. DMSO can be used to control and limit the effect of ulcers resulting from anti-cancer therapy.

Burns and DMSO

Experiments on rats suggest that partial-thickness burn wounds when treated with DMSO or DMSO in combination with other creams results in contraction of wounds. In comparison, when burn wounds were treated with silver sulfadiazine alone, the results were not as effective. One of the explanations given is that DMSO facilitates the absorption of silver sulfadiazine through the skin membrane.

There is a different class of burns called chemical burns. These result from accidental contact of chemicals and acids with the skin. In experiments with rats, an injection of DMSO in combination with other palliative significantly reduced the burn, improved tissue recovery and minimized tissue damage.

DMSO and respiration

Respiratory trauma may occur due to several reasons. In an experiment conducted on monkeys, DMSO induced respiratory response was found to be dramatic. Subsequent tests on a larger sample indicated that DMSO in combination with other drugs can enhance the respiratory response in animals. Respiratory depression has been found in humans due to excessive consumption of narcotic stimulants. Preterm babies can suffer respiratory distress due to hypoxia. When patients suffering from respiratory distress are injected with a dosage of DMSO combined with other drugs, the response was found to be significantly higher than when injected with well-known respiratory stimulants alone.

Autophagy

Cell degeneration occurs in certain disorders such as cancer and some neurodegenerative diseases. Autophagy is a term related to such cellular degradation processes. We have discussed the role of chemical chaperones in enabling unfolding of proteins. Sometimes, due to various reasons these chemical chaperones do not perform the task as desired. In such circumstances DMSO has shown great potential in acting as chemical chaperones.

Use of DMSO in animal husbandry

DMSO seems to be a favorite of horses and dogs. Reports have been published regarding effect of applying DMSO to inflamed regions of dogs and horses. Currently two DMSO veterinary products have been approved in the US.

Horses are often exposed to injuries especially in their leg and foot region, resulting in swelling. These have been treated with DMSO products. Eye infections resulting from fungus have been successfully treated with DMSO in combination with anti-fungal agents.

Pain management with DMSO

Pain can be, well, very painful. It can cause severe disability and can directly impact on the quality of life. Pain caused due to injury can disrupt normal life. Untreated tissue wounds can become infectious and sometimes become gangrenous. Healing takes time and scarring of tissues is a common outcome. Such delirious effects can be obviated with the use of proper medication.

Pain can be an adamant customer and do not respond well to local application of medication. It may be noted that DMSO has not been used directly at the wound site.

In a study conducted on rats, application of DMSO at the wound site resulted in pain relief as compared to placebo recipients. The results point to the possible use of DMSO in humans for controlling pain.

Disorders related to stomach and intestines

Most of the intestinal disorders are accompanied by inflammation to the affected area. Though management of inflammation has been well documented, not much information is available on the direct use of DMSO in managing gastrointestinal inflammation

Use of DMSO in managing Crohn's disease has shown encouraging results. The treatment with DMSO in one such study resulted in improved renal function when introduced early. Later stage intervention with

DMSO, when renal function was severely impaired showed insignificant response.

Chapter 3 - Autoimmune disorders and DMSO

To appreciate the role of DMSO in relation to autoimmune system requires a basic understanding of the autoimmune system and related diseases.

What is an autoimmune disease?

An interesting concept was discovered which linked our own body to the genesis of a disease. Our body has a natural immune system which stops our body from getting infected. Due to various reasons, this immune system attacks its own body mistaking it to be an alien or unknown bacteria or virus.

Obviously our autoimmune system goes for a toss and we become our own enemy. The guard becomes the thief by mistake. When this happens, the body sets up a defense against the foreign invaders. The defense mechanism makes proteins or antibodies which start fighting against healthy tissues. This reaction can be dangerous or even fatal in certain circumstances.

The cause of this abnormal behavior is not exactly known. However there is enough evidence to show that it has hereditary roots. Women are likely to face autoimmune diseases twice as much more than men. Autoimmune diseases are also more prevalent among certain ethnic groups. Research in this field has picked up pace lately. It is speculated that disturbance to the autoimmune system may also be caused by external agencies like exposure to adverse environmental conditions. Solvents and chemicals can also have a role to play in triggering autoimmune disease. Scientists are also pointing their finger at the dietary habits of people who go for fat laden ready-to-eat food brought directly to the dinner table from the supermarket. However, no such link has been proved.

Which are the diseases directly linked to autoimmune system?

Type 1 diabetes is the first disease linked directly to a breakdown of autoimmune system. Diabetes is a condition in which the Pancreas, an organ in the body, stops producing insulin. In this condition, the autoimmune system attacks its own healthy pancreatic cells which produce insulin.

Rheumatoid arthritis is an extremely painful condition and is prevalent in a wide swathe of population. Rheumatoid arthritis mainly affects the joints resulting in soreness and pain. This autoimmune disease starts hosing its might right from an early age and can even outlive the victims.

Multiple sclerosis affects the connection between brain and body. This is a serious affliction which deteriorates alarmingly and may cripple people within fifteen years of its appearance.

Lupus is a deadly disease which affects almost all parts of the body and damages kidneys, heart and other internal organs. It causes rashes all over the skin.

Many autoimmune system diseases have been named after their discoverers - Crohn's disease, Addison's disease and Graves' disease are some common autoimmune diseases.

You have to undergo a battery of tests to uncover the exact autoimmune disease. The antinuclear antibody test provides the first clue of the existence of autoimmune disease. This may require further tests to pinpoint the exact autoimmune disease.

What is the role of DMSO in curing autoimmune diseases?

It was reported by a group of scientists in early eighties that myasthenia gravis, an autoimmune disease, may be a result of humoral immune mechanism. In this disorder the patient experiences a slow degradation of skeletal muscles. These patients can be identified in the initial stages by the loss of control of eye movement. The disease also makes the muscles of the mouth weak making it difficult to swallow and chew. It can be a life threatening disease.

Experiments were conducted on rats which were artificially induced with myasthenia gravis. It was seen that application of DMSO orally or through other mean led to a substantial decease in antibodies responsible for the autoimmune disease. DMSO has also shown to decrease painful bladder symptoms in case of lab generated autoimmune cystitis. Human related experiments have yet to be conducted in all the above cases.

Chapter 4 - DMSO in Genetics

There are numerous diseases and illnesses which can be directly linked to genetics. Treatment of cancer with radiation has many side effects. DMSO has the miraculous property of protecting animal cells from damage caused by radiation. Numerous studies have been conducted to understand the process by which DMSO provides protection to DNA strands.

Understanding DNA and its link to life

DNA stands for deoxyribonucleic acid. The structure of DNA was discovered in a dramatic fashion only some decades back. DNA is composed of four essential bases adenine (A), thymine (T), guanine (G) and cytosine (C). These put together give rise of the famous helix structure of DNA. This helix like structure preserves the essential genetic material of which our cells are composed of.

Living cells have to manufacture proteins which are essential for survival. IN living cells DNA is copied into RNA which are called messenger RNA. These messenger RNA carry information from DNA to the cell areas called Ribosomes where proteins are manufactured. These proteins are actually amino acids linked into a chain.

So far so good. As long as the process continues in a healthy manner life goes on uninterrupted. However, nothing in this world is simple. Wear and tear is common occurrence. Every living thing must die one day due to aging and DNA is no different. The DNA strands break up due to various reasons. Luckily, there are chemical processes which repair the damage. Otherwise we would all be dead by now. DNA strands can also break due to stress created by radiation and chemical degradation.

What happens when there is damage to DNA? As explained earlier, genetic information or code is only available within the DNA. In the absence of genetic code new cells cannot be formed. Therefore when the DNA is damaged due to an assault from external stimuli like radiation, new cells stop getting produced and decay of old cells leads to tissue becoming dead. This would be unacceptable position because radiation treat is constant. Therefore a defense mechanism has evolved to repair damaged DNA. Cancer and other abnormal growth form in human cells when this repair process fails.

Where does DMSO figure in all this?

Numerous studies have revealed that when the signaling pathways are affected due to damage to DNA, cancer develops. Normally, the living cell responds immediately as soon as it detects that the DNA has been damaged. Interestingly the cell response makes very effort to repair the damage to DNA but if it fails it commits suicide and causes its own death. This fatal call is made by the affected cell to protect other cells from damage. This altruistic behavior of cells actually saves us from suffering.

Therefore when the affected cells are unable to repair the DNA it results in cancer. When breaks in the double helix strands are induced, the damage to DNA is immediate. These breaks can be caused by inducing artificial radiation into the healthy cells. This break has also been associated with the abnormal growth of free radicals.

It should be noted that damage to a single strand can usually be repaired by the cells. Damage to the double strands pulls the two strands physically apart and therefore repair becomes impossible. In this situation the only solution is for the cell to cause its own death. In case even this is not possible the cells become cancerous.

Coming back to the question of cancer stem cells, these behave life normal stem cells especially its ability to produce all cell types. Cancer stem cells are therefore responsible for many types of cancers. Cancer therapy consists of radiation which has the inherent problem that it kills both healthy and cancerous cells without discrimination. Radiation therapy is accompanied by nausea, extreme tiredness and baldness. Alarmingly, recent studies show that long term chemotherapy can induce impairment to the brain. Patients suffer from memory loss and loss of cognition.

Enter differentiation therapy

What then is the alternative? Chemotherapy, as we know, is the most popular form of cancer therapy even though it suffers from dangerous side effects. The answer lies in the way cancer is treated. In chemotherapy cancer stem cells are killed or destroyed. In differentiation therapy the cancer stem cells are not destroyed but instead they are transformed into some other type of stem cell which no longer acts cancerous.

Cancer stem cells are seen to transform into some other type of cells when exposed to DMSO. Some scientists feel that this action of DMSO can be utilized for cancer therapy. It appears that DMSO disrupts cell cycle activity. In addition reports suggest that DMSO stimulates release of the tumor suppressor protein. This property of DMSO could be used for treatment of cancer. It should be noted no experiments have been conducted to conclusively establish the efficacy of DMSO using this novel approach.

However, further research and studies are certainly warranted in the application of DMSO in the field of cancer. There is a lot which needs to be done to convert theoretical concepts into practical solutions in the treatment of cancer.

Chapter 5 - DMSO and treatment of infections

Infections cause many more deaths than any other illness. The spread of Black Death or Great Plague is known to have killed an estimated two hundred million people in Europe and Asia during the fourteenth century. There are many types of infections caused by bacteria, viruses and fungi. Bacterial infections are treated either by eliminating the disease causing Bacteria or by controlling its growth. The role of DMSO in management of infections is promising. Studies have shown that a solution containing DMSO has properties to control and limit the growth of bacteria. Tuberculosis is deadly disease which has still not been eliminated from this earth. New types of Tuberculosis bacteria have now developed resistance to antibiotics. The problem gets worse when one type of resistance is transmitted to subsequent strains of Tuberculosis. This makes their treatment difficult if not impossible. This kind of Tuberculosis gets transmitted form one person to another quickly. As such, Tuberculosis is a tough nut to crack and treatment with antibiotics has to be provided for prolonged and uninterrupted period for over six months. Fatality from this infection is also not uncommon.

There are two factors which make administering of antibiotics more efficient. DMSO acts as a carrier for larger molecules than itself to penetrate cell membrane. This means you can provide lower doses of antibiotics to maintain same effectiveness. This reduces the toxicity of the antibiotics. We have discussed the BBB or blood brain barrier earlier in this book. Antibiotics suffer from an inability to cross the blood brain barrier. Patients suffering from brain related bacterial diseases, like meningitis and brain abscess, can therefore cannot be treated effectively with antibiotics. Some studies have suggested that DMSO can facilitate antibiotics to cross the blood brain barrier. However, there are many controversies surrounding this claim. The main problem which gives rise to controversy is the inability to explain the mechanism by which DMSO carries larger molecules across the blood brain barrier.

DMSO and viral infections

Viral infections can be quite adamant and try what you may, they will not go away. Infections like Herpes have been around since ages. Mention of herpes can be found in history and have been noted during biblical times. Herpes can cause damage to private parts and also the eye, skin and other parts of the body. DMSO as a mono therapy or in combination with other drugs has proven to be effective. Untreated Herpes can also lead to deadly human viral encephalitis which can be fatal. Use of DMSO as a solubilizing agent for other antiviral drugs needs to be studied since it reduces the need for excess quality of primary drugs. This in turn minimizes the adverse effect of excess use of drugs.

Chapter 6 - DMSO and brain trauma

Thousands of fatalities occur due to brain injury caused by accidents. Pioneering research in reducing and minimizing the trauma caused by brain injury has raised interest in this field. Children and

Currently the mechanism of action of DMSO in reducing trauma in brain injuries has not been established. DMSO has many therapeutic properties. It increases the flow of blood in the brain while maintaining blood pressure. It removes fluid from the brain through urine without affecting heart rate. Sodium channel activation plays an important part in brain health and DMSO blocks this activity. We have already discussed its role as an effective free radical scavenger. DMSO slows swelling of the brain in trauma cases. All these properties together and alone make it an ideal candidate for healing brain trauma.

DMSO and tissue factor

What is tissue factor? It is phenomenon connected with blood coagulation. In healthy humans and animals, blood flow is unimpeded and continuous. The blood goes about doing its job of providing important nutrients to various parts of the body. Things get upset when the body undergoes trauma or injury. Imagine that you get injured and blood starts flowing out of the affected part. Without a mechanism which stops blood flow you will dies due to excessive loss of blood. In healthy persons the blood flow is stopped when the blood forms clots. This is called blood coagulation. This coagulation happens when blood is exposed to tissue factor. It is a protein which promotes clotting of blood. But coagulation may also prove to be fatal when brain or heart injury is concerned. Blood clots in the brain can be fatal. Therefore clotting must b prevented in such cases. DMSO inhibits the action of tissue factor.

DMSO and injury due to bullet wounds

More and more people are getting killed by other people. The free availability of guns even to school kids has made the situation worse. Gun control is a sensitive topic and legislators are unlikely to meddle with it. The gun lobby is also very strong and resists any change in laws. Deaths due to bullet injuries have risen phenomenally. Obviously lots of attention is getting paid to victims suffering from bullet injuries.

Imagine the path of a bullet when it traverses through the brain. It tears through the tissues on its path and copiously spills cerebral fluid. The skull breaks into pieces which then get embedded in the brain matter. The bullet can either be lodged in the brain or may exit causing damage on the way. Brain trauma caused by bullets almost always results in death even before the patient reaches the hospital.

Patients who are lucky to reach the hospital face another ordeal. The physicians have to address numerous issues while treating such patients.

Studies have been conducted with DMSO in managing brain trauma inflicted due to bullet injury. In one such study where DMSO was compared with standard drug mannitol in treatment of brain trauma, DMSO was found to be much superior. The researchers opine that the property of DMSO to effectively manage cardiac output which often complicates treatment of brain trauma patients.

Chapter 7 - DMSO and Geriatric research

Life expectancy of human population has increased dramatically over the last century. People are living well over eighty years due to improved healthcare and modern medicines. But the question remains unanswered whether the quality of life of this aged population has kept in step or not. To add to the problem of an aging population there are reports that medical companies are working on miracle drugs which would even reverse again process. It is predicted that humans will soon live beyond a hundred years.

The aging mechanism has not yet been unraveled. Telomerase, a substance in the living cells are getting plenty of attention from scientists in Geriatric research. Scientists are also keenly looking at the effect of diet, exercise and lifestyle on the aging process. But there is no one stop solution to stop aging. It is a complex process which involves intricate biochemical processes and mechanisms.

Round worms are the center of attraction in aging research. It is a harmless worm which does not cause infection and does not have any harmful effect on human body. Why choose a worm to study aging? Ironically this small worm shares some of the properties of humans. This worm, named C. elegans is also transparent making it easy to peek into its inner working. This worm has made its entry into laboratories and is used for testing drugs which may have a direct impact on longevity. Another important feature of C. elegans is its lifespan – it only lives for fifteen to twenty days. Even an hour's increase in its longevity can translate into years for human beings. Scientists can easily add, remove or manipulate the genes and study its affect quickly. They don't have to wait for years to observe the results. DMSO has been used as a solvent with other chemicals which are identified to provide longevity. Unfortunately, in some studies, DMSO when added as a solvent did not seem to play any role in extending lifespan of the worm. Surprisingly, when administered alone, DMSO seemed to have a beneficial effect in life extension. Some studies explain the life extending properties of DMSO due to its ability to modulate gene expression. However, a lot more needs to be done before DMSO can be used generically by the human population in relation to life extension.

Conclusion

Now that you have been exposed to most of the miraculous properties of DMSO, it is time for a roundup.

Let's begin with the wonderful property of DMSO to manage free radicals. The medical community has lately shown interest in the phenomenon of free radicals. Many illnesses have their origin in the spread of free radicals. It has been found that free radicals, when produced in the body, causes damage to healthy cells. Your body organ start deteriorating and behaving abnormally when exposed to free radicals. The damage caused by free radicals is slow and therefore difficult to detect, and by the time the damage is discovered it is usually too late. DMSO is known to remove the free radicals from the body. DMSO is also known to preserve your body's natural immune system.

We have also discussed the issue of blood brain barrier. The blood–brain barrier plays an important part in protecting the brain from many diseases caused by bacteria, viruses and other pathogens. The blood–brain barrier prevents selective transportation of pathogenic material from the blood to the brain. What this means I that your brain is protected and remain free from infection. However, this also creates problems when you have to transport medicines to the brain. The brain barrier does not allow medicines to reach the brain. This can prove to be a hindrance during treatment of mental illnesses. Though smart drugs have been developed, we still have a long way to go in achieving good penetrability of drugs to the brain. DMSO has displayed the rare property to penetrate the blood–brain barrier. This property can be used to allow movement of essential drugs to the brain. A similar behavior of DMSO is its vasodilatory property. Blood flow to injured organ becomes restricted when the blood vessels constrict. DMSO can improve blood flow to injured organs by dilating blood vessels leading to the affected are.

The role of DMSO in relieving pain cannot be underestimated. The main advantage of using DMSO for pain relief is the fact that it is not habit forming. You can't get addicted to DMSO even after prolonged use. The pain relief mechanism of DMSO is different from the action of an opioid.

We have discussed the property of DMSO as a scavenger. This property comes in handy when DMSO is used in treatment of heart diseases. Free radicals are produced more copiously during heart infarction and the normal secretion of chemicals and enzymes is unable to cope with the amount of free radicals. DMSO helps in coping with excess production of free radicals during injury to heart muscles.

Another interesting property of DMSO is its ability to work as a sodium channel blocker. DMSO has shown remarkable improvement in reduction of pain and also faster healing of wounds. The healing process is quite complex. In the healing process a chemical is released by the body which though essential, must not be excessive. The balance is critical. DMSO assists in release of this chemical as well as limits the amount of discharge.

Experiments on rats suggest that partial-thickness burn wounds when treated with DMSO or DMSO in combination with other creams results in contraction of wounds. In comparison, when burn wounds were treated with silver sulfadiazine alone, the results were not as effective. One of the explanations given is that DMSO facilitates the absorption of silver sulfadiazine through the skin membrane. Subsequent tests on a larger sample indicated that DMSO in combination with other drugs can enhance the respiratory response in animals. Respiratory depression has been found in humans due to excessive consumption of narcotic stimulants. Preterm babies can suffer respiratory distress due to hypoxia. When patients suffering from respiratory distress are injected with a dosage of DMSO combined with other drugs, the response was found to be significantly higher than when injected with well-known respiratory stimulants alone.

Experiments were conducted on rats which were artificially induced with myasthenia gravis. It was seen that application of DMSO orally or through other mean led to a substantial decrease in antibodies responsible for the autoimmune disease. DMSO has also shown to decrease painful bladder symptoms in case of lab generated autoimmune cystitis. Human related experiments have yet to be conducted in all the above cases.

The role of DMSO in Genetics is significant. There are numerous diseases and illnesses which can be directly linked to genetics. Treatment of cancer with radiation has many side effects. DMSO has the miraculous property of protecting animal cells from damage caused by radiation. Numerous studies have been conducted to understand the process by which DMSO provides protection to DNA strands.

Cancer stem cells are seen to transform into some other type of cells when exposed to DMSO. Some scientists feel that this action of DMSO can be utilized for cancer therapy. It appears that DMSO disrupts cell cycle activity. In addition reports suggest that DMSO stimulates release of the tumor suppressor protein. This property of DMSO could be used for treatment of cancer. It should be noted no experiments have been conducted to conclusively establish the efficacy of DMSO using this novel approach.

Currently the mechanism of action of DMSO in reducing trauma in brain injuries has not been established. DMSO has many therapeutic properties.

It increases the flow of blood in the brain while maintaining blood pressure. It removes fluid from the brain through urine without affecting heart rate. Sodium channel activation plays an important part in brain health and DMSO blocks this activity. We have already discussed its role as an effective free radical scavenger. DMSO slows swelling of the brain in trauma cases. All these properties together and alone make it an ideal candidate for healing brain trauma.

Studies have been conducted with DMSO in managing brain trauma inflicted due to bullet injury. In one such study where DMSO was compared with standard drug mannitol in treatment of brain trauma, DMSO was found to be much superior. The researchers opine that the property of DMSO to effectively manage cardiac output which often complicates treatment of brain trauma patients.

Put together, DMSO is surely a wonder drug which has yet to find the rightful place in the treatment of various illnesses and diseases. Its use can bring down the cost of treatment and also alleviate the pain and trauma caused by illnesses and accident victims.

Impressum:

2019 Timo Schmid
1. Auflage

Kontakt: Timo Schmid
E-Mail: Timo.schmid@gmx.at
Covergestaltung: Lisa Biegemann
Coverfoto: Depositphoto

Buch aufgeführten Tipps und Informationen ergeben, aus keinem Rechtsgrund eine Haftung übernehmen. Haftungsansprüche gegen den Autor für Schäden materieller oder ideeller Art, die durch die Nutzung oder Nichtnutzung der Informationen bzw. durch die Nutzung fehlerhafter und/oder unvollständiger Informationen verursacht wurden, sind grundsätzlich ausgeschlossen. Rechts- und Schadenersatzansprüche sind daher ausgeschlossen. Das Werk inklusive aller Inhalte wurde unter größter Sorgfalt erarbeitet. Der Autor übernimmt jedoch keine Gewähr für die Aktualität, Korrektheit, Vollständigkeit und Qualität der bereitgestellten Informationen. Druckfehler und Falschinformationen können nicht vollständig ausgeschlossen werden. Es kann keine juristische Verantwortung sowie Haftung in irgendeiner Form für fehlerhafte Angaben und daraus entstandenen Folgen vom Verlag bzw. Autor übernommen werden. Solltest du nicht genau wissen, ob diese Tipps aus dem Ratgeber für dich geeignet sind, so nimm Kontakt zu deinem Arzt oder Apotheker auf.

Für die Inhalte von den in diesem Buch abgedruckten Internetseiten sind ausschließlich die Betreiber der jeweiligen Internetseiten verantwortlich. Zum Zeitpunkt der Verlinkung wurde die jeweilige Webseite auf Vereinbarkeit mit deutschem Recht überprüft. Verstöße gegen geltendes Recht wurden nicht festgestellt. Bei den verlinkten Webseiten handelt es sich um Inhalte Dritter, für die der Autor nicht verantwortlich ist. Eine regelmäßige Überprüfung der verlinkten Webseiten auf Rechtmäßigkeit kann der Autor ausdrücklich nicht leisten. Der Autor hat keinen Einfluss auf Gestaltung und Inhalte fremder Internetseiten. Diesbezüglich distanzieren sich Autor und Verlag von allen fremden Inhalten. Zum Zeitpunkt der Verwendung waren keinerlei illegale Inhalte auf den Webseiten vorhanden.

Hinweis: Aus Gründen der besseren Lesbarkeit wird auf die gleichzeitige Verwendung männlicher und weiblicher Sprachformen verzichtet. Sämtliche Personenbezeichnungen gelten gleichermaßen für beiderlei Geschlecht.

Kontakt:

Timo Schmid
Münzweg 4
9500 Villach

CPSIA information can be obtained
at www.ICGtesting.com
Printed in the USA
LVHW012017020821
694317LV00033B/2943

9 781797 536736